Pandemica

also by P.J. Reed
poetry

FLICKER

HAIKU NATION

HAIKU ICE

HAIKU YELLOW

HAIKU SUMMER

HAIKU GOLD

Pandemica

Poetry of the COVID-19 pandemic by P.J. REED

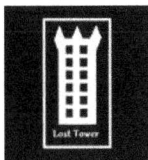

Lost Tower Publications

Pandemica by P.J. Reed

published in 2021

by Lost Tower Publications

ISBN-13: 978-1-80068-298-6

Pandemica

Preface
Generation COVID

Sometime in spring 2019 normal life changed. For years the World Health Organisation had been ringing alarm bells, the 'once in a century' pandemic was late. In the past, this was true, the Spanish Influenza Outbreak of 1918 and the Great Plague of the Middle Ages ravaged unchecked around the world, killing millions of people. However, with the technological advances of the twenty-first century, a pandemic seemed impossible. After all, international medical efforts had contained the West African Ebola virus epidemic and the SARS outbreak (Sudden Acute Respiratory Syndrome) and kept deaths from these epidemics to the thousands. The international medical response to these disease events showed how well-equipped governments and health agencies were to respond to evolving diseases.

However, nature is an organic entity.

She changes and evolves.

It was as if these earlier disease outbreaks were testing our medical defences, searching for the ways in modern life which made us vulnerable to modern disease. After years of exploring, nature found our weakness – we had the technology, lines of communication, and ability to stop diseases reaching pandemic proportions, our weakness was not technology but our very nature.

The hidden numbers of deaths in Wuhan, China and the suppression of people and social media sources that warned of the new SARS-like virus created a false picture about the severity of the new virus.

In the early days of the virus, international borders remained open. People travelled for business and pleasure, and super-spreaders spread the disease wherever they wandered.

As COVID entered each country through ill-timed holidays or business trips, governments implemented their pandemic containment policies.

A total of eleven pandemic/epidemic exercises were carried out in Britain between 2015 and 2019, including Exercise Alice in 2016, which tested Britain's readiness to cope with Middle East respiratory syndrome, caused by a coronavirus.

Firstly, people with symptoms of the virus were isolated and people they had been in contact with found and given tests to prevent the virus entering the local community. However, too many people were in contact with other people and the house isolations became community isolation bubbles, in an attempt to stop the virus passing from community to community. Still the virus spread. As each containment policy failed, COVID-19 spread to every corner of the country and on 26 March 2020, England went into a national lockdown with the Prime Minister, Boris Johnson ordering the population of England to stay at home.

Supermarket shelves emptied, vegetable seeds disappeared, and toilet roll mountains grew inside people's homes as fear descended.

We had become Generation COVID.

A Note From The Poet

Pandemica is the poetry collection I never expected to write. Who thinks they are going to spend a couple of years, basically under house arrest, while a deadly virus, which some people still don't believe exists, rips through the world population? It definitely falls into the realms of science fiction and to be honest I don't write that sort of poetry. However, when science fiction became fact, I thought I had better put pen to paper or fingertips to keyboard and start recording the pandemic.

This collection is a personal account of the pandemic, how it affected people both local and internationally. It is a record of the triumphs and ebullience of the human spirit in times of adversity.

Often it is the little things that see people through such times which are then forgotten, their importance lost. Such as the nation-wide Thursday night 'Clap for the NHS' on your doorstep. A time when people could step out of their houses and wave to their neighbours and hear the whole of their hidden community coming together as one beating saucepans, clapping, and cheering, all in their own little household bubble.

Children at home, their schools closed indefinitely painting rainbows, their parents taping them to front windows to bring a message of hope and thanks to the key workers who continued to work throughout the pandemic.

People shopping for their elderly neighbours they barely knew before the pandemic, or shops and restaurants delivering food to their customers. This collection is about the 'ordinary' heroes of the pandemic such as the Tiverton egg woman, who sold eggs from her chickens in a wooden box at the end of her garden, so people would not have to risk catching the coronavirus by shopping in town.

This collection is also a celebration of family.

A 'thank you' to the one member of each family deemed the strongest and healthiest, who risked death and disease by doing the weekly grocery shopping.

It is about the army of grannies who were called upon in the early days to rip up their sheets and make homemade facemasks for everyone they knew, even though the facemasks, made of three layers of cotton sheets were like breathing through cardboard and were replaced as soon as possible.

It is a celebration of parents who, while working from home, became teachers and mental health specialists overnight, as well as foragers, rifling through emptying kitchen cupboards but still magically creating meals for their families every day of the lockdown.

Pandemica is also a memory of Friday night quiz nights – when random groups of families came together to do quizzes together over the once unheard of 'Zoom' video communications in place of pub visits and meals out. It is the family sitting around the television in silence listening to the Prime Minister unveil the latest COVID restrictions and having a cup of tea and any available biscuit to recover from the news.

Finally, *Pandemica* is the voice of the unknown people, living through extraordinary times.

A Review

Haiku is an ancient Japanese poetry form, whose origins date back to the Edo period. It is a mirror on the human condition describing people and their actions in succinct, minimalist detail. *Pandemica* is a combination of the formal haiku and senryu poetry styles and their direct opposite, that of free form open poetry. In this way, P.J. Reed has been able to explore the COVID-19 pandemic both as a series of captured moments and memories as the haiku style dictates, and as a descriptive narrative of events, as free form poems allow.

Throughout the unfolding disaster of the pandemic Reed has recorded the lives of the 'ordinary' people, exploring their actions and emotions, and has captured a snapshot of their life in verse. Thus, creating a fascinating representation of the triumph and tragedy of human spirit in a time of adversity.

P.J. Reed is mainly known for her seasonal haiku collections which are written in traditional Japanese haiku and senryu. Each of these poetry styles consists of three sections, where the first and last lines contain five moras, while the middle line has seven. The mora is a unit of sound in the Japanese language.

Unfortunately, due to the dissimilarities of Japanese and English language the formal writing of haiku and senryu has had to be adapted. Moras cannot be translated into English and therefore syllables are used in their place. Syllables are the nearest equivalent to moras, in Western language. Consequently, formal westernised haiku is written as seventeen syllables divided into three lines of five, seven, and five syllables.

Another difference between Japanese and westernised haiku is in the physical line structure of the poem. Haiku can be written in one or three vertical lines in Japanese, whereas in English the poem is divided into three horizontal lines.

Apart from the obvious differences in written structure, the actual essence of haiku and senryu has remained the same bridging both cultures. Traditional haiku does not rhyme or contain punctuation and has a juxtaposition, or cutting word, on the first or third line dividing the poem into contrasting parts. Haiku is usually written with natural and seasonal references with feelings and thoughts succinctly captured in one breath.

Senryu developed from haiku. Haiku was seen as a poetry form for the elite. While senryu was viewed as verse for the masses and became especially popular among the working people from the eighteenth century onwards. It was named after Karai Hachiemon who wrote senryu under the pen name Senryū or River Willow.

Senryu has a similar physical construction to haiku but where haiku dwells on aspects of nature and always contains a *kigo* or season word, senryu is a written commentary on man and the manmade. It can be comic, cynical or darkly humorous, a comment on human predicaments or human emotions. One example of the comic nature of senryu, can be found in Karai Senryu final verse which stated -

> write me down as one
> who loved senryu,
> and loose women

In *Pandemica*, P.J. Reed has taken the comic and satirical origins of senryu and reintroduced them into a pandemic setting, two deliciously biting examples being,

businessman panics
face masked and suffocating
while his wife walks on

hanging from an ear
his facemask swings in the wind
protecting his chin

Reed has also explored on the darker places, which people experienced while living through the pandemic with commentaries of fear, loneliness, and disease –

a child in the park
runs to greet her long lost friend
stops six feet apart

the conspiracy
a nurse replaces vaccine
killing with saline

Reed's open form poetry juxtaposes well with the bravery of her senryu, creating deeper insights into the pandemic world, with her beautifully emotive, descriptive narratives. Whereas her haiku and senryu are written photographs of COVID-19 her open form poetry present as films chronicling life in full colour. I particularly enjoyed her intense narratives of the lives of individuals during the COVID-19 pandemic, many of which have been made into spoken word short films.

This book is a captivating ride through the troughs and peaks of humanity in crisis.

A monumental read.

by Karen Jones

Index of Poetry

Contents

Poem number	Title	Page
	The First Lockdown	
1	containment circles	19
2	COVID in the wards	20
3	Humanity In Absentia	21
4	Humanity Paused	22
5	Lockdown Life	23
6	Rumour Nation	24
7	Parklife 2020	25
8	dog owners' pockets	26
9	Rainbows and Fevers	27
10	Twenty-Twenty Fashion	28
11	rows of just living	29
12	propped upon pillows	30
13	Shops	31
14	a child in the park	32
15	grabbing toilet rolls	33
16	human exhibits	34
17	old man walks home	35
18	reports of dying	36
19	fractions have arrived	37
20	life shifts to cyberspace	38
21	COVID statistics	39
22	a nurse sits and cries	40

The Second Lockdown

23	Lockdown Part Deux	42
24	an angry binman	43
25	return to lockdown	44
26	businessman panics	45
27	Covid test results	46
28	crunching through gold leaves	47
29	eat out to help out	48
30	Astra Zeneca	49
31	silent salsa hall	50
32	vaccine party time	51
33	Chest tight breathing hard	52
34	flesh-coloured facemasks	53
35	hanging from an ear	54
36	pandemic faux pas	55
37	queuing by the bank	56
38	twenty-twenty left	57
39	Tits On A Beehive	58
40	Locked Down	59
41	unusual sounds	60
42	Return To Parklife 2021	61
43	The Return	62
44	a sudden heatwave	63
45	the mid-morning break	64
46	of masks and glasses	65
47	time traveller comes	66
48	COVID family	67

The Third Wave
Freedom Day Postponed

49	captive and maskless	69
50	freedom postponed	70
51	appointments only	71
52	pandemic rages	72
53	the disappointment	73
54	the conspiracy	74
55	social bubbles popped	75

Freedom Day Arrives
Welcome To the COVID
World

56	Generation Millienia	77
57	Excuses	78
58	Freedom Day	79
59	nightclubs reopened	80
60	vaxer refusenics	81
61	parents' dilemma	82
62	Gen X	83
63	his final words were	84
64	ping isolation	85
65	injection nation	86
66	the fear has fallen	87
67	COVID-19 Appitude	88
54	A Masked Response	89
55	Pinged	90

56	eyes itch chest restricts	91
57	summer festivals	92
58	Cornwall in flames	93
59	Death Of A Radio Host	94
60	test cricket cancelled	95
61	final COVID days	96
62	petrol shortages	97
63	home unremedies	98
64	first cold of autumn	99
65	government warnings	100
66	travel restrictions	101
67	ghost of Christmas past	102
68	two years of COVID	103
69	Omicron moments	104
70	The High Street	105
71	twenty-twenty two	106
72	the bearded lady	107
73	Spawn of COVID	108
74	COVID Cloudfall	109
75	The Empty Chair	110

Of Poetry

The History of Haiku	112-3
Glossary of Terms	114-5
How To Write Haiku	116-7
Bibliography	118

The First Lockdown

containment circles
Leicester under COVID dome
still cases increase

COVID in the wards
no face masks or green gowns left
nurses wear aprons

Humanity In Absentia

Blue skies cover cities
mountains pierce through
once polluted clouds.
Ozone hole resewn.
Rivers run clear
deer sunbathe as
wild boar roam
and pumas stalk
the emptied streets.
Earth trembles less,
footprints are swept
away by summers
soft breeze.
Humanity in absentia.

Humanity Paused

Sometime in March
the world stood still,
humanity placed on pause.
Faces masked and scarved
as sanitized hands slowly dried
and a million people died.
Open borders closed their gates,
land bridges failed to land.
Houses labelled 'social bubbles,'
sat with gates chained shut.
Summer journeys went unwalked,
as corona bought a first-class ticket
and flew across the world.

Lockdown Life

Morning
Duvet trapped
I cannot escape

Bulging freezer
Dominies on
Speed dial

Morning spent
Unwrapping
Virtual box sets
On Netflix

And repeat.

Rumour Nation

It came from out of China,
an unwanted Wuhan takeaway
with a free fortune cookie,
number four, corona to go.

It leaked out from a bat lab
playing pass-the-virus-parcel
as, suddenly sick, its scientists
silently faded from this world.

It was invented by the pharma,
big companies bored with cancer,
decided to create instead of cure,
a new virus, pandemic for a profit.

It's a governmental conspiracy,
to control the unkempt masses,
with unknown viral terrors, and
confine people to their homes.

Parklife 2020

There are more children
playing in the park,
than at the school next door.
They watch through railings,
wash hands, use porta loos,
packed in their classroom pods.
The 'Stay-at-Home' heroes
sunbathe in the park.
Kids bikes whoosh wildly
round on muddy tracks,
eat dusty snacks with dirty hands,
savouring their freedom.
While furloughed fathers
teach football skills
and wildflower names,
and teenagers sit cross-legged
in segments of a social circle,
two metres from their friends.

dog owner pockets
searching for a crumpled mask
will a poo bag do

Rainbows and Fevers

Stay at home heroes
dig for victory
carrots grow in old paint pots
potatoes planted in plastic bags
We make do and mend.
Dock leaves forest on uncut verges
wildflower roundabouts bloom
Careless talk costs lives
unsocially we distance
two metres from humanity
coughs and sneezes spread diseases
We chat to unknown neighbours
through peeling back garden fences
while rainbowing front windows
and clapping for our lives
corona sends no warning.

Twenty-Twenty Fashion

Furloughed families
in daytime pyjamas,
support the NHS.
Stay-at-home heroes
draw rainbows and clap,
bang on saucepan lids
while social distancing
among manicured gardens,
in little family bubbles and
annoy the night-time workers.

They listen to daily briefings
watch 'R' rate rise and fall
in this pandemic waltz.
Scurrying to the open shops
in homemade PPE.
Old floral sheets and
ugly, unused scarves
wrapped tightly around
sweating faces
and fogging glasses,
in twenty-twenty fashion.

rows of just living
attended by white suits with masks
pandemic patients

propped upon pillows
he breathes through a flexitube
wide eyes full of fear

Shops

Solitary shops stand
sparkling, shining,
in the winter showers,
surrounded by a sea
of empty spaces.
A silent tsunami washed
the High Street shops away.
Their greying husks
rain-soaked and worn,
stand steadfast, resolute
watching, waiting,
for the passing of the storm.

a child in the park
runs to greet her long lost friend
stops six feet apart

grabbing toilet rolls
he weaves through the empty shelves
clutching precious haul

human exhibits
hidden under glass and brick
nature has been freed

old man walks home
plastic bag full of food tins
rests and rubs sore hands

reports of dying
the new Wuhan takeaway
a global franchise

Pandemica by P.J. Reed

fractions have arrived
parents claim that maths has changed
Descartes shakes his head

life shifts to cyberspace
virtual cafes and coffee
phone calls left unheard

COVID statistics
Daily global spreadsheets scream
Data bytes of death

a nurse sits and cries
everybody is dying
thirteen-hour shift

The Second Lockdown
31st October 2020

Lockdown Part Deux

Locked in on lockdown
part two, the sequel,
storyline copied, character
development minimal.
Actors look slightly drunk.
Threat level is unchanged
and plot holes unplugged.
The audience is confused and
the ending unsatisfactory.
Sequels always suck.

an angry binman
discussing second lockdown
a load of bullocks

return to lockdown
social life unaffected
a book is opened

businessman panics
face masked and suffocating
while his wife walks on

COVID test results
ominous red line appears
health bar subtracted

crunching through gold leaves
discussing toilet closures
two angry women

eat out to help out
support your local café
corona-to-go

Astra Zeneca
called in with the weak and old
thought I was healthy

silent salsa hall
becomes a vaccine centre
would prefer to dance

vaccine party time
heart and head pound in rhythm
eyes refuse to see

chest tight breathing hard
corona is not like flu
misinformation

flesh-coloured facemask
the shop assistant's mistake
a horror feature

hanging from an ear
his facemask swings in the wind
protecting his chin

pandemic faux pas
a leopard print facemask
knickers on her nose

queuing by the bank
COVID safe and masked in black
hostile withdrawal

twenty-twenty left
under bursting COVID cloud
new year new COVID

Tits On A Beehive

Wailing sounds arise
from beneath the shaking bedding,
seeking sanctuary in the sheet fort
that covers the once living room
now transformed into an
algebraic battleground.
She f-ing hates home schooling -
'Everyone can just ask Alexa
and 'x' can bloody well stay lost.'
I warn her that such language
is not appropriate for school and
nor is throwing furry-faced slippers
at the home school prefect.

Perhaps 'Maths Monday' was not
my best idea, I flap a white hanky,
pass a peace offering through
the closed, pegged door as our
children run round screaming
in impromptu creative play.
When I ask if she will continue,
once our enforced lock-in ends,
a head appears unsheeted,
hand gripping a mug of wine-
'I'd rather cover myself with honey
and staple my tits to a beehive
than f-ing home school our kids again.'

Locked Down

Comfort food filled bellies
bulge over jeans shrunk
in washing machines.
Drooping pyjamas are
your new workwear.
Back garden benches
for quiet mugs of tea,
sit in front gardens
waiting to catch slow
moving neighbours.
Puberty waves once more
with face mask rashes
and exploding cheeks.
Flowerbeds turn to
vegetable plots and you
realise if society collapses
your one surviving
carrot will not last long.
While you scurry face hidden
masked and hatted into
newly opened hairdressers
and having to admit you
cut your hair and yes
it's harder than it looks.

unusual sounds
screams and giggles fill the park
children have returned

Pandemica by P.J. Reed

Return To Parklife 2021

Pink blossom confetti
blows across the park.
Leaf streamers hang
on pondside willows
now lying duckless
as the people return.
Enclosed, the playground
bursts through its bars,
swings soar screaming,
through the morning air.
Mummy's sit in circles,
clutch paper coffee cups
watch wobbling toddlers
race on worn ride-on toys,
tailwaggers bark cloudward,
watch screaming sealess
gulls feed greying chicks.
Parklife has returned.

The Return

The park smells of aerosol
And springtime blossoms,
As man sprays white lines
Across the green field,
And the footballers return.

a sudden heatwave
sunglasses and flower masks
the world seems misty

the mid-morning break
Bourbon biscuit tastes of tin
she prefers cocoa

Pandemica by P.J. Reed

of masks and glasses
with each breath a fog descends
patients disappear

time traveller lands
he realises his mistake
and abruptly leaves

COVID family
everyone is positive
grandma is missing

The Third Wave
Freedom Day Postponed
June 2021

captive and maskless
found on sticky toilet floor
my blue surgical mask

freedom postponed
COVID cases surge once more
odd face tans remain

appointments only
book online or through the phone
twentieth in queue

pandemic rages
general practitioners
missing in action

the disappointment
government sanctioned hugs
are now permitted

Pandemica by P.J. Reed

the conspiracy
a nurse replaces vaccine
killing with saline

school bubbles popped
mass isolation broken
COVID unchained

Freedom Day Arrives
July 2021
Welcome To The COVID World

Generation Millienia

COVID restrictions lifted,
Masks off, bars open,
Boobs bandaged, chests waxed,
Skirts raised and muscles bulged
Player ready for kicks and giggles,
Parties in the summertime-
And self-BBQ's on the beach,
While bodies ripple in the clubs,
Pornstar Martinis in one hand,
Selfie-machine in the other.
Generation Millennia unleashed.

Excuses

Fifty thousand new cases,
The R-rate lies forgotten,
Resting in trampled pieces
As the COVID wards refill,
Mortality rates are climbing
Among the vulnerable and the old
But their deaths lie uncounted
as they would die soon anyway.

Freedom Day

Freedom day arrived
Along with the Delta variant
Fifty thousand cases
Pretend they don't exist.
Masks off, if you want,
Legs out, if you like,
Summer is in flames,
Variants are waving,
Don't burn your mask just yet.

nightclubs re-opened
slow dances and fast kisses
COVID partied hard

vaxer refusenik
declares his faith will save him
taken by COVID

parents' dilemma
COVID or the new vaccine
which will hurt their child

Gen X

Generation X-cluded,
brought up alone, ignored,
unattached to the amniotic cloud,
parents unavailable, lives detached.
but they knew the rules:
if it's still attached it's fine,
eating dirt will make you strong,
come home when it's dark,
but don't disturb your father.
Generation X-trema
brought up on tight leather,
big hair, and alpha male
post-apocalyptic madness,
the children of the popcorn,
ready for the food wars to begin.
Four million deaths and rising.
They bulk buy seeds and flour
just in case society collapses
and the undead come at dawn.
Generation X-orcist
they were made for this.

his final words were
I wish I'd had the vaccine
death of a sceptic

ping isolation
confined to house health arrest
running low on cheese

injection nation
a gateway drug to concerts
and dirty dancing

the fear has fallen
people smile as they pass by
greetings are exchanged

COVID-19 Appitude

Download the app,
turn on your Bluetooth,
scan in each QR code.
The blue app will track you
through the day, recording
paths upon paths,
intersections unwelcome,
potential vector exchange plotted.
Your compliance is required.
Log in your life, your
vaccination information,
report any sudden symptoms,
record your COVID tests and
remember we are tracking you

A Masked Response

Unmasked and unafraid,
a customer, almost naked, chooses
tuna melt over five cheese toastie
and spies a plague propaganda victim
timidly cruising the sandwich counter
fogged glasses peering over a surgical mask
'Living in fear, huh!' he comments
 angry hands squeezing his panini flat.
'Yes,' said tomato and mozzarella panini guy
'I work with the young, elderly, and sick
and I don't want to kill anyone,'
the doctor, seven years in training, replies.

Pinged

The mobile pinged, too loudly,
a vibrant alert in monochrome
of tornado warning stature.
it was not my chosen chime.
My phone had been invaded,
altered by agencies unknown.
It beaconed, pulsed, and glowed,
in warning shades of red,
security had been compromised
invaded by an alien, origin unknown,
possible exposure, only six days ago,
now called to isolate and protect
those free from pathogens
who I spoke to yesterday.

eyes itch chest restricts
leaves fall as allergies rise
people run past fast

Pandemica by P.J. Reed

summer festivals
loud music and free COVID
gift from BoardMasters

Cornwall in flames
a corona staycation
catch it if you come

Death Of A Radio Host

He researched fully-
on Facebook and Goggle,
in search of logic and common sense,
away from governmental hysteria,
he found that his odds of dying
were way south of one per cent.
He was right, COVID was just like flu
governments and scientists were wrong
he grabbed his rights and stood firm
against the rise of the nanny state,
he was the voice of reason
then he caught corona and died.

test cricket cancelled
an Indian camp outbreak
stumped by corona

final COVID days
on oxygen and TikTok
posts final message

petrol shortages
empty supermarket shelves
the yoghurt has gone

home unremedies
take bleach or some worming pills
and wear a beak-shaped mask

first cold of autumn
hacking cough and feeling hot
PCR says no

government warnings
another year of COVID
need to buy more wool

travel restrictions
the Omicron variant
is already here

ghost of Christmas past
as families ungather
frozen turkey laughs

two years of COVID
still unable to work out
which face part to mask

Omicron moments
latex clinging and brow sweating
fears spacemen are next

The High Street

Shop assistants work
behind glass cages,
masked and muffled,
but still the battle rages.
Triple-boosted we roam,
Protected? Yes...maybe,
but many stay at home.
As dead shops peer
through smashed windows
a stopped clock, an unticked tock,
circa mid-pandemic lockdown.
Open doors and windows,
but meeting outside is safer.
We watch the news and wait
to reclose once more.

twenty-twenty two
or twenty-twenty part two
life stuck on repeat

the bearded lady
she strides along the high street
black mask around her chin

Spawn of Covid
Covid – the gift that keeps on giving.

It's what they don't tell you
 that matters. Congratulations
you survived the hacking cough
burning body and much more,
but what they don't warn you
on the scribbled scripts or TV Ads,
is that the spawn of Covid will be
coming back for you. An insidious
little creature, playing hide and seek
with your soul. It will squeeze your lungs,
and churn your brain, turn your
taste bud dials to zero, cranks
your temperature gauge to full
and stab sharp pins into your legs.

It is the Spawn of Covid
and will be your friend for life.

COVID Cloudfall

The COVID cloud descends
Secretive, fog like with
fever dreams and compacting breath.
I heard a man cough last week,
hacking over his maple hazel latte.
It might have been COVID or a reaction
to a face full of whipped cream.
I blame him not the cream.
Now I'm sick after two and a half years COVID free
I thought I was immune.
Unfortunately, I was just lucky.

The Empty Chair

The armchair sat vacantly
Staring at the TV
Not right at the screen
Straining to catch every muffled word
But neatly in chair formation
With our packed settee
The cushion in perfect tassel alignment
With its fellow furnishings
The chair sat patiently
Ready to be filled
Not knowing you were gone.

Of Poetry

The History of Haiku

Haiku is an ancient Japanese artform dating which originated from the Heian period of Japanese culture (700-1100). In this period, it was a requirement of polite society to be able to recognize, recite, and participate in *renga* or collaborative, long poetry writing activities at social events and lavish house parties. *Renga* was one of the most important literary arts in pre-modern Japan. The verses used sound unit counts of five-seven-five and seven-seven and finished with two lines of seven sound units each. At this time, poets considered the use of *utakotoba* as the essence of creating a perfect *waka* and use of any other words were considered unbecoming of true poetry.

A *hokku* was the opening stanza of *renga*. It had a special status in the poem and was written by the host or a guest of honour. A *hokku* was composed of seventeen moras or sound units broken into phrases of five, seven and five sound units respectively. Alone among the verses of a poem, the hokku included a *kireji* or cutting word which appears at the end of one of its three phrases. Like all Japanese writing it was written vertically down the page and not horizontally as in western writing.

In the sixteenth century, with ongoing military conflicts within Japan and the eventual rise of the Tokugawa shogunate, Japanese poetry underwent a mini revolution becoming freer and less complicated.

By the time of the great *haiku* master Matsuo Bashō (1644–1694), the *hokku* had begun to appear as an independent poem and was also incorporated in *haibun* (a combination of prose and *hokku*), and *haiga* (combining a picture with a *hokku*). In the late 19th century, Masaoka Shiki (1867–1902) renamed the individual *hokku* poem *haiku*.

A traditional *haiku* poem has three lines, where the first and last lines contain five moras, while the middle line has seven. The *mora* is a unit of sound in the Japanese language, which is the Japanese equivalent to a syllable, but it is not the same. *Moras* cannot be translated into English and therefore syllables are used in their place. When westernized, *haiku* is written as seventeen syllables divided into three lines of five, seven, and five syllables.

Traditional *haiku* does not have a title, rhyme, or contain punctuation but they have a juxtaposition on the first or third line dividing the poem into contrasting parts. The *haiku* is usually written with natural and seasonal references with feelings and thoughts succinctly captured in one breath.

Glossary of Terms

Haibun	A combination of prose and haiku.
Haiga	A picture combined with haiku.
Haijin	The writer of haiku.
Haiku	Haiku is a highly structured form of Japanese poetry. In western culture haiku is easily recognisable from micro-poetry by its structure. Haiku is made of three lines. The first line contains five syllables, the second seven syllables and the third five syllables. Traditional haiku must contain certain elements such as a *kigo* and a seasonal element. It consists of a moment in nature captured and recorded.
Haiku Moment	The intense focus on one moment in time. To capture and freeze that image in haiku before it is lost or altered by the passage of time.
Hokku	The original form of haiku. The opening stanza to a *renga*. A long poem written by many people as a form of entertainment for the ruling elite of Japanese society.
Juxtaposition	When sentences are placed together with a contrasting effect.
Kigo	A word that implies the season of the haiku.
Kireji	A cutting word that denotes a break between the two parts of the haiku when writing in one-line Japanese poetry. There is no English

114

	equivalent to this although some poets may put a dash in their haiku to denote the change.
Koan	A *koan* is a Zen Buddhist contemplative phrase which contains a logical contradiction or paradox, designed to challenge the reader.
Mora	The *mora* is a unit of sound in the Japanese language, which is like a syllable, but not the same.
Sabi	The innate loneliness of life.
Senryu	A form of human haiku, expressing emotions or human actions. It has the same structure as haiku but does not have to contain a cutting word.
Syllable	A syllable is a single, sound unit of a word.
Tanka	A *tanka* is similar to haiku but consists of five lines and thirty-one syllables. Each line has a set number of syllables see below
	Line one – five syllables
	Line two – seven syllables
	Line three – five syllables
	Line four – seven syllables
	Line five – seven syllables
Utakotoba	Words suitable to be used in songs or poetry.
Wabi	The austere and severe beauty of nature expressed through writings of spiritual solitude.
Waka	Traditional Japanese poetry.

How To Write Haiku

Everyone has their own writing style, and it is always important to let your writer's voice come through into your writing. However, some poetry is defined and recognisable by its external structure such as two-line Erdo love poetry, which as its name suggests has to contain two lines. Similarly, a sonnet is easily recognisable for consisting of fourteen lines written in iambic pentameter, while a limerick consists of five lines, written in a predominantly anapestic meter and have a strict rhyme scheme of AABBA. Likewise, traditional haiku has its own distinctly recognisable structure of three short lines. The first line contains five syllables, the second has seven syllables, and the last line consists of five syllables.

In the beginning, it is hard to contain your writing and thoughts within the narrow confines of haiku.

I tend to think of haiku writing as playing a game of chess. It requires practice, strategy, and mathematical precision. As with any skill, haiku thought needs hours of practice to attain, but with practice you will develop a way of thinking that automatically responds to the five-seven-five syllable scheme, which is immediately recognizable throughout the world as haiku.

I find my best haiku writing moments are away from people just walking with my dog, or alone and watching nature without the hindrance of man. I have been asked by several passersby what I was doing, as I stood and memorized the mechanics of a droplet of water falling off a leaf. One man even stopped his car in a lane to find out the reason behind my unusual behaviour. In these situations, it is always better to reply that you are writing haiku and not in fact watching a leaf. One response will get such replies as 'very noble' and 'how exciting,' the other will get you a sideways glance and a wide berth.

Once I have observed an event and the tingling of a haiku begins to form, I try to write it down as soon as possible. Normally, when I write a haiku, the picture or memory is written within the first two lines of the haiku. The juxtaposition comes in the final line and will be either a comment on the picture formed, an extension of the image to other areas, or even what happened afterwards. For example, what happened to the leaf or droplet of rain after it had fallen. So, while the last line is still related to the first two it is obviously different.

Sometimes, when trying to write a haiku, it will not conform to the correct structure. However, a haiku should never be forced. It should be a natural extension of a scene. If the poem you are writing is either too big or too small to fit into the exacting haiku structure just accept that it is not going to be a haiku and write a poem or micro-poem instead.

Finally, the most important part of writing haiku is to have fun and not take it all too seriously.

Bibliography

"The Serious Side of Senryu," Edited by Alan Pizzarelli, Simply Haiku: A Quarterly Journal of Japanese Short Form Poetry. Autumn 2006, vol 4 no 3

"Senryu | Japanese Poem," Encyclopedia Britannica. N.p., 2016. Web. 27 Dec. 2016.

"Senryu: Refreshing The Human Spirit". Haiku North America. N.p., 2016. Web. 27 Dec. 2016.

"Simply Haiku: Quarterly Journal of Japanese Short Form Poetry – Showcase," Simplyhaiku.com. N.p., 2016. Web. 27 Dec. 2016.

"Some Senryu About Go," Kiseido.com. N.p., 2016. Web. 27 Dec. 2016.